THE
HAPPINESS
SWITCH

How to transform anxiety, depression and other negative moods by focusing on and cultivating good feelings

CHRISTINE ELLIS

This book is not intended as a substitute for the medical advice of physicians. The reader should regularly consult a physician in matters relating to his/her health and particularly with respect to any symptoms that may require diagnosis or medical attention.

The Happiness Switch
Copyright © 2016 by Christine Ellis.

All rights reserved. Printed in the United States of America. No part of this book may be used or reproduced in any manner whatsoever without written permission except in the case of brief quotations em- bodied in critical articles or reviews. This book is a work of fiction. Names, characters, businesses, organiza- tions, places, events and incidents either are the product of the author's imagination or are used fictitiously. Any resemblance to actual persons, living or dead, events, or locales is entirely coincidental.

For information contact:
Christine Ellis
http://www.findgoodfeelings.wordpress.com

Book and Cover design by Christine Ellis
ISBN-13: 9781540640208
ISBN-10: 1540640205

First Edition: September 2016

10 9 8 7 6 5 4 3 2 1

CONTENTS

THE HAPPINESS SWITCH I
FOREWORD 1
PART I: 6
INTRODUCTION 6
WHAT THIS BOOK IS ABOUT 7
WHAT THIS BOOK IS NOT 10
MY STORY 12
PERMISSION TO FEEL GOOD 21
PART II: 24
THE METHOD 24
O V E R V I E W 25
ON BROCCOLI AND RUNNING 32
(TO PUT IT A DIFFERENT WAY) 32
THE STEPS 37
STEP 1: TAKE YOUR EMOTIONAL TEMPERATURE 38
BE SPECIFIC: NAME THE FEELING 43
STEP 2: ASSES YOUR CURRENT STATE'S EMOTIONAL CHARGE 48
STEP 3: CULTIVATE THE CLOSEST POSITIVE FEELING YOU CAN REACH FOR 52
THE WORKINGS OF THE EMOTIONAL TRAMPOLINE: BOUNCING FROM THE NEGATIVE TO THE POSITIVE 59
DEALING WITH THE RESISTANCE TO CHANGE 70
A BRIEF RECAP 76

THE HAPPINESS SWITCH

IS THIS A CURE? 78

PART III: 81

EASY DOES IT (AND WHY IT IS REALLY, REALLY, REALLY IMPORTANT THAT YOU DO!) 81

1. A CAUTIONARY TALE 82

2. BABY STEPS 88

4. PUT ONE FEELING BEFORE THE OTHER 92

PART IV: 95

LIVING THE GOOSE BUMPS 95

1. CULTIVATE POTATOES BEFORE YOU MOVE ON TO ORCHIDS ...96

2. A DAILY PRACTICE 99

3. "BUILD IT AND THEY WILL COME". 103

CLOSING WORDS 106

APPENDIX A 108

APPENDIX B 126

ABOUT THE AUTHOR 130

PLEASE REVIEW 131

Foreword

"I do suffer from depression, I suppose. Which isn't that unusual. You know, a lot of people do." **Amy Winehouse**

THIS IS A BOOK ABOUT WHAT I LIKE TO CALL "THE DUMPS". I like that umbrella term because it covers all sorts of stuff, from the blues that you can't shake away, to the days when you can't get out of bed, all the way to the panic and anxiety you feel at the thought of never having X thing or person you think are absolutely necessary for you to FINALLY be happy.

I had a bad case of "the labels" for a very long time: depression, anxiety, moods... the list can be long.

Now I just call it all "the dumps". I make the whole thing smaller. It is also a whole lot less important – and it has much less power over me.

THE HAPPINESS SWITCH

I will use just one more label, to throw it at you for the simple reason that I want you to know that I have been there too and I know you can come out the other end.

I've had PTSD. The long label is "Post-Traumatic Stress Syndrome". If you are not familiar with this one, they give it to war veterans, rape victims and others who receive such shocks to their systems that they can't seem to recover.

It's depression and anxiety with the extra kick – nightmares, panic attacks, night sweats, social isolation, dissociation, high anxiety, mood disorders… all rolled into one.

I've had that, even though I've never been in a war or raped. But I have experienced many shocks to my system and at some point I just couldn't get back up.

I will tell you more about my story later. For now, just know that I HAVE gotten back up – and then some.

I have discovered a way of being in my head, all the time, that:

- makes me healthy, joyous and content.

- that allows me to enjoy my relationships and be fully present for those I love and who love me.

- that kicked procrastination in the teeth and got me back to chasing my dreams. Not only chasing them, in fact, because when I got back I was actually much wiser and stronger, so I started making my dreams happen.

So now I'm writing about my journey. I'll show you how I did it – and what I do every single day.

I know it works. No drugs required, nor therapist – though both can be useful and I am the first one to encourage you do get the help you need.

This book is for you if you:

1. have struggled with "negative emotions" for a long time (fear, desperation, frustration, discouragement, sadness etc.)

2. feel like you have no power over the negative emotions – or you simply don't know how to change them

3. have tried various healing modalities and, while they have all made you feel better, you couldn't find one that "stuck

4. have been told, or tell yourself that you "feel too much

It's a funny thing about that last one, by the way – people say you feel too much only when it comes to the "negative" feelings. Nobody ever says it about joy. Like "Oh, you are feeling way too much joy!"

This is what we will talk about here: feelings and moods.

I will teach you:

- How to generate good, positive feelings at will

- How to stay in good feeling states, moods and feelings consistently

THE HAPPINESS SWITCH

- How to coach yourself out of "the dumps

Believe it or not, you are your own best guide.

Do you know why?

Because nobody can feel for you! Meaning, of course, nobody can feel feelings in your place.

No matter how much they want to help, you must find a way to come to peace with, change and harness your feelings.

Until you learn to do that, you will not find your thriving life.

Material stuff and "big breaks" don't work all that well either.

Don't you know people who seem to have it all but are incredibly miserable and even self-destructive?

I waited for a long time for the "big break" to come thinking that THEN I will be happy.

So the break came and I STILL wasn't happy.

That's when I shook myself up, gathered all the wisdom, wits and knowledge I had and finally did it.

I did it for love, really. I would like to say that it was for myself, but it was (at least at first) for my family. Because I love them so much and I wanted them to live with the healthy, happy version of me. Perhaps you relate to that.

I hope you will find your own motivation for healing. I'm just here to share how I've done it –and hope that it will inspire you to do it too.

Part I: Introduction

What this book is about

THE HUMAN MIND HAS LONG BEEN LIKENED TO A GARDEN. Wise men tell us to cultivate good thoughts and weed out the bad ones. Indeed. It is the highest of practices.

High it may be. But easy, it is certainly not.

Learning how to cultivate good feelings and transform the negative ones is not exactly what we learn in school. It is not even something that a lot of us learn in our families, or society at large.

"Oh, you have the blues? Just put on some happy music."

Or:

"When I'm afraid? What I do? (smile) I just pretend I'm not!"

THE HAPPINESS SWITCH

And so it goes...

We sort of take these things we call "feelings" as they come and we hope the bad ones avoid us like car accidents and the flu. If we do "get hit", well... each person is different. There is no recipe here for how we deal with the bad feelings, although a few common threads emerge: drugs, alcohol, shouting, bad relationships with others, insane abuse towards self...

Winston Churchill used to call his depression "The Black Dog". The dark feelings hounded and chased him his whole life.

Perhaps you feel the same way.

Maybe you have tried talk therapy, drugs (legal or not), self-help and aromatherapy. Massages, cognitive therapy and EFT (Emotional Freedom Technique). And more.

At the end of the day – or, better said, after a while, the feelings came back.

If you feel like this describes you, you are in the right place.

I struggled with these issues for years.

I am a regular person plagued by a traumatic past that left deep wounds. I tried to heal them in so many ways – and they all helped, of course. But there always came a time when I would "fall back" into my old ways. I was back on the treadmill.

I will tell you more about my own story in a little while.

For now, what I want you to know that I have discovered a way of managing my feelings that allows me to snap out of anxiety, depression and other "Black Dog" feelings and transform them into the goose bumps feelings.

Does it take a bit of work? Yes.

Is it easy? Much easier than you think.

Does it last? If you work it, it does.

Is it quick? Yes. If you work it.

It's a bit like dieting. If you've been eating junk food for a long time, you can't expect to run a marathon the first time you eat an apple. You understand that you must make changes in your diet – and your lifestyle – and that these changes take time.

The method I've worked out for myself does this with feelings. I will teach you how to put "good feelings" in your system and transform the bad ones.

In time, the Black Dog will become a puppy. You won't be afraid of it anymore and it will not dominate you every time it shows up. You will live in the sunshine and you will know what to do when the "negatives" show up – as they will, as they are a part of being human.

This is what this book is about.

What This Book is Not

IN THIS BOOK I WILL TEACH YOU HOW TO TAKE HOLD OF NEGATIVE FEELINGS and transform them into positives.

But this is not intended as a crisis manual. If you feel that you are in great suffering, please ask for help! Seek a counselor or a doctor.

Acute pain needs to be tended to – and you cannot get that from a book.

Also, I am a regular person who, after years, of struggle, has discovered something that works in dealing with anxiety and depression. But I am not a medical doctor.

I am not denying, in any way shape or form, the value of

therapy, medical help or any healing modalities. Rather, this method is meant to be complementary to them.

My Story

THE SUN WAS FILTERING IN THROUGH THE LEAVES OF THE TALL TREES IN OUR BACK GARDEN. I could see a squirrel effortlessly jumping up thin branches. Beyond the terrace, the forest was peaceful and serene.

I could feel the couch under my body. Its leather stayed cool and comfortable even with the heat.

Our beautiful home was filled with the laughter of my perfect little boy who was pushing toy cars around with his father in the upstairs office.

I really had everything I had ever wanted. I had found my home, my family and my life. Things had never been as good as in that moment and I knew that they were going to get even better.

So why was I not happy?

Another question: why was I afraid to be happy?

Or another: why was I allowing fear to steal from my happiness? But how could I stop it? It was everywhere. Fear that it would all go away. Fear that something was going to happen to one of us. Fear that the sky would fall on those tall and strong trees and on the little squirrel.

I hated the struggle. I hated the dark feelings. I wanted with every fiber in my being to feel good, to inhale the happiness that was clearly in front of me.

That was the day I turned a corner. That was the day when I said to myself: "If I don't learn how to be happy now, under these circumstances, I never will be."

* * *

When I was 7 years old, my father got very sick. I witnessed his struggle with cancer and then his death, three years later.

After his passing my mother fell into a profound depression. She would sit for days that turned into years on her bed, smoking cheap cigarettes and crying.

If I went to ask her how she felt, she would wave me away. "Just go," she'd say. "Go away."

So away I went, to my room and to my books. I was already carrying in my belly the struggle and the darkness.

THE HAPPINESS SWITCH

We had no money. There was one year when we ate boiled potatoes for Christmas.

I lost the innocence and the joy of childhood very early on.

Already at the age of eight or nine I was plagued by deep feelings of insecurity, loneliness and despair. Life was truly bleak.

My young adult years were not very happy either.

I often gave my power away to abusive relationships and situations. I gave up quickly on the good because I did not feel that I deserved it.

Throughout the years I tried to find solutions to my profound unhappiness.

I read a lot of self-help books and tried several approaches.

At some point I even saw a psychologist, on and off, for two years. I was diagnosed with PTSD – Post-Traumatic Stress Disorder. It was "official": I was constantly living in fear.

All of these explorations were useful... up to a point. I would get better for a while and then... I would fall back into my old patterns.

The pull towards unhappiness and misery was so strong that it was very easy for me to go back to that place. And for a long time I could not find a solution that would "stick".

Until that day when I was sitting on the couch at home,

watching the garden and listening to the sounds of my happy house.

I had been married to my wonderful husband for more than two years. I was the mother of an incredible little boy. I had the perfect home. And I should have been happy. But... even though I had moments of happiness, I was still plagued by profound fears.

I had nightmares. My anxiety had begun to spike up again, on a daily basis. I wanted to be a writer but I was blocked and stuck.

You see, I had always thought that "One day, when I get my life in order, THEN I would be happy."

I was waiting for the magic, perfect time when I will have gotten everything I wanted.

And here they were: my wonderful moments had come, I was living my wonderful life... and I could not FEEL how wonderful it was.

So that day, sitting on the couch in our living room, it finally dawned on me that it had become a habit. It was ingrained, stuck in m bones like muck on the plumbing of the house.

I was stuck on anxiety, fear, anger, misery, bitterness and the likes. The only thing standing between me and my "wonderful life" were these very feelings.

The outside conditions of my life should have given me those feelings! And they had... for a short while. But then I fell back into my habits of feelings that I had been "practicing" for decades.

* * *

That day I decided to just take one good feeling and focus on it. Not something big like enthusiasm or joy or excitement, but something more low-key. I decided on "calm". I liked "calm". It was doable, achievable and it didn't deny the fear either. There was no struggle. Calm it was.

I could see the trees outside our home with their refreshing green leaves gently swaying in the wind. There was calmness in the trees.

Then I thought about other things that evoked the feeling of calmness: a quiet afternoon at the beach; a good meal; watching a good movie... I just stayed with that for a little while... and felt better. Just thinking about "calm" began to settle it inside of me a little, without me trying to do it so.

It was a sort of "watching a feeling" play out in the world. Not necessarily in my world, but out there too, in other people's lives, in the past or in the future.

So I left it at that.

And I tried again, the next day.

All the years of therapy, self-help books and healing methods had taught me this though: easy does it.

By then I was wise enough to take small steps and not jump

high into those high-octane feelings like elation or victory. Nothing "top of the world". Just simple, modest, day-to-day goodness, calm, curiosity, wonder, comfort, simplicity or relaxation.

I "watched those feelings" every day, in my mind's eye, like a sort of contemplative meditation that could be done in front of the kitchen sink or pushing the shopping cart at the grocery store.

There it was, the word of the day: simplicity – appearing in the clean lettering of the pickles jar and the mother wiping her child's nose.

I started feeling better more of the time. My moods stabilized.

I began to do the "watching the good feelings" thing throughout the day.

Whenever I felt a pang of fear or anxiety, I would try and think about calm or contentment or simple curiosity.

I didn't think about enjoying my life, feeling wild happiness or love or bouncing off the walls with the pleasure that should have been mine. I just... saw the good and cleanliness in washing the dishes; the softness of my baby's hair; the calmness in my husband's breathing.

Ordinary life, indeed, is not so ordinary after all.

Slowly I began to turn things around. Not only were my moods more stable, but I could actually enjoy more of my

THE HAPPINESS SWITCH

life: my moments with my son and my husband, our life together, our home, my friends and all the other blessings I had.

After a few short days, an email came in. A friend was inviting me to join her new business venture – custom-made for me, creative and inspiring.

Another few weeks and I ran into a book that cured my procrastination. I started writing again – and drawing.

Blessings came knocking on my door. None of them earth-shattering, but I didn't need that kind of drama anymore. I was simply happy with my everyday miracles of well-being and finally feeling the blessings all around me.

I had finally found "the switch".

* * *

I was truly amazed. This really worked. And I hadn't even tried to MAKE something happen. I had simply wanted to FEEL the bounty in my life.

How ironic and heartbreaking that I had gotten there but could not feel it...

But I had finally figured it out for myself – the way to be present, to be there, to "think positive thoughts".

Contemplating these good feelings is a practice I have since deepened and that has brought me the healing that I had been looking for.

In a way, I recognize all the teachings that I have absorbed rolled into it. Now I understand all of them better. Perhaps I had simply not "clicked" with them before.

Now that I have… it seems so simple and so obvious. But then, everything is – in hindsight.

Do I still have bad thoughts? Sure. Am I "cured"? I don't know… I still struggle sometimes. But I know what to do. I cultivate good feelings. And my mental garden is growing beautiful and strong – just like my life.

* * *

So this is my story and this is how I came to live this process that I will teach you in this book.

It is a very simple one. It uses something that you do every single moment: feel.

You will not need anything on the outside of yourself – except, perhaps, pen and paper so you can write out your thoughts and emotions for better clarity and to enhance the process.

You will not be required to take any action. In fact, it is better if you refrain from taking ANY action, at least for a little while, until you get the hang of it.

THE HAPPINESS SWITCH

Feelings are magical. They are beautiful in and of themselves. And, cultivated in and of themselves, they bring blessings unimagined.

I couldn't believe it before I saw it. But now that I have... I can tell you first-hand that it works, that depression and anxiety are not a life-long sentence and that, indeed, light can brighten up even the darkest corners.

Permission to Feel Good

I don't know about you, but for a long time I struggled against feelings as if they were gods: creatures outside of me, with a mind of their own, whose will or whimsy could make me or, most of the time, break me without my consent or willingness.

For the longest time I seemed to have little power in affecting any real change into my mood.

Much like everybody else, I believed that outside circumstances determine in large part the way I felt.

If my life was going well, I felt (sort of) good. No problem there. Except… in my life there were plenty of times when the outside circumstances were quite terrible – and so were my feelings.

THE HAPPINESS SWITCH

In rare moments I had glimpses of joy or relief when my mind said that I should not feel those things at all, given what was happening. It seemed sacrilegious.

I was around eight years old, to give you one example, when my father came home from the hospital where he was being treated for cancer, to find me happily bouncing off the walls because I had been to a friend's birthday party. He thought my joy was indecent. I should have been more aware of his suffering.

I felt so ashamed by my joy that I put it out immediately, the way you would a fire. And not only for that particular moment, but for a long time.

Celebrating, really celebrating, felt wrong to me for decades. What if there was someone sick and suffering near by?

Or how could I allow myself to thrive and feel strong when, after my father's death, my mother fell into a terrible depression? She paid no attention to me for a couple of years afterwards – and everybody else seemed to think that this was okay AND that I should be doing the same thing: cry all the time.

I know that these are highly personal examples… some of you will agree with one side of the story, some with the other. But I think that everyone will understand the point that I am trying to make:

At some point, we who learned to feel bad on a regular basis stopped giving ourselves permission to feel good.

Long after a bad situation ended, we continued the mourning. We stayed low. We kept our head down and our moods in the dumps.

I did it out of loyalty and compassion for my parents. I did not know any better at the time and I did not understand that by dampening my own well-being I wasn't helping them anyway.

It took me a very long time to overcome this... and I am not sure I will ever be "completely cured". I will still feel a little bit guilty here and there. But I have learned to give myself permission to feel good, enough to start thriving.

Do you think you could too?

Nobody else outside of you will ever be able to do it.

Part II:
The Method

Overview

THE SIMPLEST WAY TO DESCRIBE THIS "GOOD FEELINGS METHOD" IS THIS:

1) choose a feeling you want to feel (not related to a specific situation, person or set of circumstances)

2) cultivate the positive feeling of your choice by thinking of people, places, things or situations that evoke that feeling for you.

That's it. At its most basic level, this is all it takes.

I can hear you grumbling though. I know I would have, a few years ago. It would go something like this:

Aha... sure... you mean to tell me that, first of all, I can choose how I feel? Ha! Yeah right... good luck with THAT! And secondly, I don't understand the part about "people, places, things or situations that evoke that feeling". What does that have to do with my specific problems? How is that going to pay MY rent? It will only make me mad, because I'll be bumming around all day in my head, thinking about what, lollipops and rainbows? Get REAL!

I will explain it all in the following chapters. For now, let me assure you that yes, you actually can choose how you feel.

But I agree with you: there is a trick.

YOU CAN'T HAVE VERY STRONG NEGATIVE FEELINGS ABOUT SOMETHING AND TRY REALLY HARD TO FEEL A POSITIVE FEELING WHILE LOOKING AT THAT SOMETHING.

It would be like trying to imagine you are eating chocolate while there is actually a spoonful of week-old leftovers in your mouth.

No, of course you cannot do it.

But you CAN feel whatever feeling you want, IF you don't try to apply it to certain situations or people.

You <u>can</u> and surely <u>will</u> feel the curiosity of a little boy standing in front of a store window, if you look at HIM; you can and surely will feel tenderness if you think of a grandfather caressing the hair of his granddaughter; you can and surely will feel contentment if you think of how someone must feel at the end of the perfect vacation day.

So how is this going to help me with my problems? you ask.

Here I have make quite an important confession: I don't know exactly how it works. All I know is that it does.

First of all, you will have the immediate benefit of feeling better, because instead of swimming in soul-twisting feelings and moods, you will (and very quickly, actually) start running positive feelings and states through your system.

Someone might argue that this, in and of itself, is the goal, the reason why we do everything we do.

People take drugs in order to feel ecstasy. Imagine being able to conjure it at will, without the aid of any physical substances (other than the ones that already exist within your body or that your body is able to produce, like dopamine).

But, of course, we want specific things, specific situations and specific feelings.

We want our problems to go away, because we think that they are the reason why we feel that bad.

If you stay focused on good feelings long enough, your problems WILL start to mysteriously dissolve.

One logical explanation is this:

By focusing more on these "pure good feelings" you actually start vibrating more and more of the time on their wavelength.

You build your good-feeling muscles, which become stronger and stronger with each passing moment, until one day you look at your former problems and they just don't seem so big anymore. They don't evoke the same feelings of helplessness, rage, indignation and so on.

Another way of putting it is this: if you have been starved of nutritious feelings for years, you can't expect to have the strength and stamina to run a marathon. You might barely be able to go to the grocery store.

But once you start eating well (putting those "good feelings" in your system) – and consistently so – you begin to get stronger. Then you have much more power to deal with your life.

<u>The other explanation</u> for why focusing on pure feelings works in solving specific negative situations is this: **pure positive feelings have, just like electricity, magnetism that is generated by the current that flows through them.**

They are, quite literally, attractive and they "pull in", just like magnets, whatever vibrates on the same wavelength – nice people, all kinds of comfortable things and situations, all kinds of beautiful things, situations and people and so on.

Feelings are attractive in nature. Because they are vibration, they will "reverberate" – or vibrate together – with everything on the same or near-by wavelength.

It is much like a radio signal – and you are the one emitting it!

I am sure you know the snowballing effect that anger has... you start getting pissed-off at someone and then you start remembering not only what they have done to you recently, but everything they have ever done to wrong you. And it's not just them... it's other people too! Now you are disappointed with people... and afraid that you will never find true friends... or your soul mate...

One thing leads to another. "Like attracts like" indeed.

You don't have to apply those good feelings to specific situations in your life.

In fact, it is better that you don't even try, because you are very used to thinking about those specific situations in certain negative ways. Trying to pretend otherwise will only make you feel worse.

It WILL feel fake to you and this is why you might be thinking "Oh, this positive thinking stuff is bs."

> *Practicing just "feeling good" by contemplating **pure good feelings** will not only make you stronger but **it will spill over into everything else**.*

I am sure you have noticed that whenever you fell in love. When you are walking around in the high of love's first blush, everything seems to come together: money comes to you unexpectedly, strangers smile, traffic is better and the radio seems to be playing your favorite songs all the time.

THE HAPPINESS SWITCH

It is a weird sort of thing... but the better it gets, the better it gets – everywhere in your life!

Good feelings will have their own snowballing effect.

For example, "calm" will "call in" other emotions which are in its vicinity, like "serenity", "peacefulness" and "contentment".

And some of these emotions will even have just a little bit more in them, which will make you feel even better.

For example, "contentment" resonates with "calmness", but it also resonates with "pleasure", which is more than "calmness".

"Pleasure" resonates with "contentment", but it also resonates with "excitement"!

Thus is the power of feeling good!

Conversely, when you are trying really, really hard to hammer good feelings on situations and people who don't evoke them from you, you actually accomplish the opposite: you reinforce those bad feelings.

You are literally contemplating "angry", "disgusted", "fed up", putting them in your system so to speak, feeding your emotional body those negative feelings so how can you possibly make "contented", "joyful" and "strong" grow in you on top of that? It's just not possible. Those circuits are jammed.

I have already hammered this point in several different ways, but it is worth repeating one more time.

When you first begin, it is very, very important that you focus on these pure good feelings.

Don't defeat yourself before you see results by trying to solve the problems in your life. Just learn to simply feel good again.

If you don't attach your problems to the good feelings, you will see that not only you CAN feel good, but it is quite easy! It is easy to do it and easy to maintain it – for days, weeks, months or years!

Later on, when you get stronger and the practice of feeling good is becoming second nature, you can tackle specific problems too. But it will be different. You will have ways of looking at things that you cannot possibly imagine now.

While doing the practice of learning to feel good feelings again, situations will have resolved themselves as if by magic. Your life will start to work out in strange ways indeed.

Just give it a bit of time.

Start small and just learn to feel good again.

On Broccoli and Running (to put it a different way)

IMAGINE THAT EARLY ON IN YOUR LIFE YOU WERE FED SOMETHING quite bad for your health. Not bad enough to kill you, but bad enough to make you sick – but only a little.

You didn't think much of it at them time, because you did not know any better. You took it and ate it and somehow got used to it. So used, in fact, that it made you sick for a long time but you didn't pay attention anymore. You thought it was your "normal".

You suffered from this low-grade fever which is called

depression, with different temperatures like anxiety, despair, self-hatred and hopelessness.

The moment came though when you began to notice that you are not in the best of health.

Perhaps the healthy parts of you that still functioned properly were sending signals that something is wrong.

At your core, the strong current of health and well-being was sending powerful messages: "You are NOT thriving! This is NOT normal!"

So perhaps you began to look into it.

For many of us, this is the beginning of a long process of healing that feels like being thrown in the deep end of the pool without an oxygen mask – and you cannot really swim.

We struggle and struggle for a long time. It feels suffocating.

The thrashing and the struggle feel better than the poison though. We simply know we MUST do SOMETHING.

So the first thing we usually do is turn back and try desperately to find out where and when the poison started coming into our system.

Now, does it seem to you like this is a useful exercise?

How can that counteract the effects of the poison? The years of suffering?

You can drive yourself crazy trying to follow this line of

thought – and keep yourself more miserable, probably for years if not decades. And now it is not because of the poison, it is because you don't think you should have been given the poison to begin with – and you don't know the antidote.

I get it. I really do. It is a very appealing thing to do, because we think that once we get to "the culprit", we will do two things: 1) make them suffer really badly, for what they've done to us and 2) pulverize the poisonous food into the ethers.

With "emotional food" though it doesn't quite work that way.

You may indulge your urge for vengeance and look at the poison as much as you'd like – but that will NOT get you the nourishment that you need.

How is looking at the weeds on your plate make broccoli appear?

It won't.

So what do you do instead? You go look for broccoli!

You know it is out there, somewhere.

You can at first look at it from a distance, then get yourself a little closer until, at last, you can have it on your plate.

The food analogy is not quite perfect though because, unlike food, emotions "end up on our plate" immediately.

> *Just starting to look for kindness "out there in the world" makes you feel it instantly – thus, nourishing you.*

It is, in a very real sense, on your plate.

Of course, this does not mean that it will be there ABOUT A PARTICULAR ISSUE, as we have already discussed. It may spread itself there anyway, as time goes on. But it may not.

You might be able to learn to feel joy, curiosity, fun, tenderness and glee again. Just not about your nasty former teacher or school bully, to give you a couple of random examples.

In time though, and if you persist, you will build a life based on joy, curiosity, fun, tenderness, glee and much more, aside from your nasty former teacher or the school bully or any other "poisons."

They will become very small in comparison to all the goodness that will flow. So small, in fact, that they will be inconsequential.

I will shamelessly mix metaphors here and say that you will learn to stretch your emotional muscles again – and run wherever you want in your life, regardless of what you have been through.

It is irrelevant whether you failed to run a marathon when you were 3, or 9, or 15. Now you get to do it your way, you get to go wherever you want and with whomever you want – and

THE HAPPINESS SWITCH

as fast as you want.

And it all starts with getting your emotions in order again – and learning to direct them at will.

One other thing is worth saying though: just like with broccoli or running, at first it will taste and feel awkward.

If you've been on a steady diet of very-bad-for-you chips for years and sitting glued onto a couch, eating broccoli AND running won't feel so awesome at first.

But they will feel BETTER.

The lessons to draw here are:

a) you need to keep at it

b) things will start building up and

c) give the process the necessary time.

The Steps

Step 1: Take Your Emotional Temperature

FEELING IS SOMETHING WE ALL "DO", ALL THE TIME. It's like breathing. You cannot turn it off.

If you are alive, you feel.

We have already established that if you picked up this book, you haven't been feeling that well.

I am willing to bet that this not feeling all that well has been going on for quite some time.

Whatever event (or events) started the chain of pain for you may long be gone from your experience, but its effects are still spilling over in your life.

Children are generally happy creatures. Have you ever seen a depressed baby?

We come into this world bursting with life and joy and if nobody messes it up for us, we carry on with our explorations, bubbling on and finding our natural balance of what we need, what we want, what is available and what we can make available through our dreams and efforts.

But if we are messed with, we change. The strong current of life energy gets pinched off.

The balance gets tipped from us feeling good most of the time, to us feeling "bad" – and I am using quotes because that is an umbrella term for a whole range of negative feelings of different intensities.

What makes the matter even more complicated is that this happens at a time in our life when we are much too young to have developed our emotional vocabulary.

We cannot put words to our hurts and we do not know how to undo them.

So the emotional wounds fester and we get this low-grade fever called "anxiety and depression".

If this is left untreated for a long time, you may even begin to think that you have lost the ability to feel good at all.

THE HAPPINESS SWITCH

You may be able to force a little smile here and there but you can't remember the last time you felt genuinely carefree or happy.

If I were to ask you "What emotions do you feel, most of the time?" you would probably groan and just say "Bad, horrible, depressed, disappointed..." Only a few words.

In a way, it seems even terrible to describe it in more detail because it is like an exercise in twisting the knife in the wound.

But naming feelings has a way of releasing the pent up energy behind them.

Haven't you ever felt this? When you felt something bubbling in you, a torrent of energy searching for an outlet and then, suddenly, you burst: "I feel damned sad and angry!". It IS a release.

Years of feeling "bad" give us the wrong perception that feelings are something to be afraid of.

With the mind of a child, who does not have the skills for dealing with it, anger seems huge. It is dangerous to feel it because mommy and daddy will probably be angry back.

Sad is huge too, because it points to a loss and we do not know how to make what was lost come back again.

But we lose something in the process: our very life. We do not blossom with the same richness that we sense exists underneath it all. Not because we do not have the words for the feelings, but because we do not have the feelings – the bad AND the good.

I have discovered in my own life that I had been focusing on the bad feelings way too much. I had been dissecting them, observing them, cataloging them and wearing them on display on my sleeve, so to speak, in the proverbial heart.

But that was because I did not know what to do with them.

Then, in the process I have described in the beginning of this book, I discovered that they are not all that powerful.

Negative feelings are natural reactions to certain life situations. The problems begin when they fester and take over parts of a soul.

I used to believe that, in order for the bad feelings to resolve themselves, I needed to process them.

It wasn't very clear to me what this processing meant exactly... but I went with the common belief that you go to a shrink (a nice one) and you sit on the couch, telling him or her the stories of your life.

Well, I processed. And processed. For a couple of years – with the therapist. On my own, I "processed" for decades.

But guess what... at the end of it all, I was still stuck in the same atmosphere that my problems had created. I was still ruminating. My feelings didn't "resolve themselves".

I still had the same question that popped up regularly (and by that I mean every day): "What do I do in my head every

THE HAPPINESS SWITCH

second and every day?"

All the years of "processing" never taught me how to actually feel good.

It is assumed that feeling good comes naturally after we "process".

Perhaps it works for some people... It didn't work for me and I have never met anybody for whom it has.

And, by the way, I am not criticizing therapy here. I do believe that it is a necessary and immensely useful way of treating soul wounds.

I would, however, add to it this very useful life skill: learning to feel good again, instead of assuming that it will happen naturally.

When you learn to replace negative feelings with positive ones, when you develop new and good feelings habits, you stop being afraid of the negative feelings. They don't hold power over you anymore, because you know what to do with them.

Be Specific: Name the Feeling

THIS SUB-CHAPTER IS ABOUT NAMING SPECIFIC FEELINGS: the negative feelings like dissatisfaction, bitterness, anger and so on and the positive feelings like giddiness, fascination and excitement.

I have included it for two reasons:

1) it might be useful to know where you are, in order to determine where you want to go.

In other words, finding ways to assess where you are in terms of emotions, beyond simply "bad".

THE HAPPINESS SWITCH

Why is that necessary?

We rarely think of emotions as goals in and of themselves.

We have no problems envisioning a college degree, a car or an apartment as the end goals.

But feelings? Whoever decides to write "joy" on their vision board? A wise man or woman, that's who.

Because "joy" is the final destination anyway – it simply takes different shapes and forms.

When we feel frustration though, joy is a million miles away. When we feel depressed, joy is a hundred million miles away. But even in frustration or depression, we can understand the opposite side of the coin: satisfaction and happiness.

So learning to name feelings will come in as a useful exercise in learning to "flip the coin": jump from "sad bad mad" to "glad good kind".

2) the second reason I have included this chapter is to help you expand your emotional vocabulary

Have you ever tried to write down all the positive feelings that you feel on a regular basis? How long do you think the list is?

My guess is that it will be pretty short (a dozen or so).

How about the list of good feelings that you know of? This one will probably be a bit longer – but not by much.

There are hundreds of words that describe emotions. Some overlap. But they all bring extra nuances of goodness. Some bring a whole lot of it

So back to being more specific with your feelings…

Taking our own emotional temperature is something that we do all the time, actually. We are self-assessing our emotions constantly. You may not realize that you are doing it but think about it: how many times in a day do you have fleeting thoughts such as "Oh this feels good!" or "Eeeek, that sucks!" or "I'm not feeling great right now…" to more defined emotional words such as "Angry!!! I am mad as heck!" or "I'm so disappointed…"

We don't pay that much attention to all that. It becomes as ingrained as dealing with bodily functions. Do you feel the urge to pee? You go to the bathroom. You get angry? Find someone to yell at.

Obviously, if we are swimming in happy emotions there is nothing to do other than enjoy them. Well, we could perhaps think of ways to enhance them. And we can surely think of ways to have them more often.

But if we are struggling with your moods, if you are swimming in the murky waters of pain, it might be useful to take your emotional temperature on purpose, to learn to describe it and assess it beyond "bad" and "painful".

Why? To find a new direction – the opposite of THAT.

This is not an exercise in stirring pain.

THE HAPPINESS SWITCH

Because the next step will be to flip it around.

If you know you are feeling angry, you may want to choose patient or understanding or wise from your emotions palette.

If you assess your emotions and you discover frustration, you may want to head towards contentment instead.

If you carry "unworthy" in your bones, you may want to cultivate the opposite feelings of "important", "unique", "interesting" or "valuable".

In the next section I will show you how to cultivate feelings on purpose.

But for now, please go to the back of the book, to **Appendix A**, which contains a list of both negative and positive feelings.

Study the list.

Then do the following exercise, which I call an "awareness exercise". The reason you do it is to bring something to your conscious awareness. In this case, your habitual emotions.

AWARENESS EXERCISE #1

CONSCIOUSLY, PURPOSEFULLY STOP AT LEAST ONCE DURING YOUR DAY TO ASK YOURSELF: "HOW ARE YOU FEELING?" AND THEN PUT A WORD TO IT.

For now you don't need to do anything else. Just get in the habit of asking yourself how you feel on a daily basis –

hopefully more than once.

One other thing: don't get too distracted by the very long list of "negative" feelings. They are there to bounce off of but not to wallow in them.

It helps to have a long list of toxic substances – and their antidotes! – just in case you have a problem. Just don't sniff them on purpose.

So: "How are you feeling?"

Ask yourself that – and give yourself an honest answer.

You do NOT need to do anything about it at this point – which, you may discover, is quite a relief.

We often jam ourselves up emotionally because we are trying to get out of a "bad feeling" but simply looking at the feeling without the need to do SOMETHING about it is, in and of itself, quite liberating.

Do this for a few days, at the end of which we will start to define your very own emotional vocabulary even further.

You will see which emotions (bad AND good) you feel regularly and you will maybe have a few surprises with some feelings that were there but, undetected and un-named, managed to slide by.

This is the emotional pool you are swimming in right now.

Before we make some changes to it though, there is one more, very important thing to discuss: feelings have different emotional charges.

Step 2: Asses Your Current State's Emotional Charge

I HOPE THAT YOU HAVE DONE THE EXERCISE in the previous section, which was to simply stop during the day and ask yourself "How are you feeling?" then giving a specific answer with the name of a specific feeling.

If you have been doing this for a few days, you might start to notice some patterns. Maybe you already know them ("Oh yeah, I'm angry all the time. So?") or maybe you are discovering some interesting things ("Hm... my DESK makes me feel whaaaaat?").

Conversely, perhaps you have been discovering that you do feel some good feelings every once in a while, like curiosity or interest. Nothing major, like passion, enthusiasm or excitement, just a few, small stirrings of life-giving positivity.

I hope that this exercise will have revealed to you two things:

1) your current emotional landscape, better mapped and named

2) the wide variations of feelings and their intensities.

Which brings me to a very important point that we need to discuss, before we talk about making the shift, on purpose, from negative feelings to positive ones:

FEELINGS HAVE DIFFERENT EMOTIONAL CHARGES

Feelings have different intensities.

Not all "bad" feelings are equally bad and not all "good" feelings are equally good.

Despair is much "heavier" than loneliness. Excitement is much more "charged" than curious.

I am using the word 'charged" because in feelings there is a certain flow of energy or power, similar to electricity.

We all intuitively sense the different intensities in feelings.

People even have natural inclinations towards a certain "emotional charge".

We sense whenever a person is naturally calm and another just "born wild".

See if you can do another quick awareness exercise.

AWARENESS EXERCISE #2

Look again through the list of feelings, both good and bad, in Appendix A.

There are hundreds of feelings so you don't need to do the whole list. Just skim through it and try to do the following exercise:

As you read through the list of feelings and feel drawn to certain ones, put a number next to them that describes the strength of their emotional charge, on a scale of 1 to 10.

In other words:

1= not very strong

10 = very powerful

For example, "despair" would be a 10 for me. "Frustration" would be a 6. "Boredom would be a 2" (it is a negative feeling but, at least for me, it is not very strong. I know I can change it very easily).

Please go ahead and do this now. It is very important!

***

Alright. Have you done it? Great! Now let's move on to how you can actually do an emotional turnaround: how to shift from a negative state to a positive one.

Step 3: Cultivate The Closest Positive Feeling You Can Reach For

SO FAR WE HAVE EXPANDED THE EMOTIONAL VOCABULARY beyond "good and bad" and we have also talked about the fact that feelings have different charges to them.

There is one more thing to do before I show you how to turn a negative feeling or mood into a positive one: **learn how to cultivate a feeling on purpose.**

What I mean by "cultivate" is really very simple: look for any situation, person or thing, imaginary or real, which evokes that feeling in you.

Let's say that you want to feel **contentment**. Ask:

"What does contentment mean to me? When do I feel it? When do other people feel it? When do animals feel it?"

You might think of someone taking their morning coffee on a sunny terrace. Or a cat purring on its owner's lap. Or the perfect fountain pen that you had in 5th grade.

There are no right or wrong answers and everybody is unique so my answers would certainly be different from yours.

But the purpose of this exercise is not to be right or wrong. It is to evoke a certain emotion, in a pure way.

The PURE way simply means that this specific emotion is not attached to a particular goal of yours, or a particular situation.

Here are a few more questions to illustrate this point:

Where does "giggly" show up? Who is giggly? When were you giggly? Can you imagine a situation in the future when you will feel that?

THE HAPPINESS SWITCH

You are like a life detective, looking for these feelings in action out there in the world – and in your world.

And will this make me feel giggly? you say. Or excited... or comforted...

It actually will.

If you don't believe me, just try it. Think about a feeling and how and where it shows up in the world for only one minute and see if it doesn't start rubbing off on you.

Feelings are contagious.

Boredom and anger are contagious. So are joy and enthusiasm.

I am convinced that you have experienced that. But you have probably experienced it without any say in the matter: you walked in on someone who was angry or bored, or joyful and enthusiastic and simply "caught" the feeling.

It works.

So why not work this on purpose and for your own benefit?

Feelings CAN be cultivated on purpose.

It is a new way of looking at the world and for me it was completely revolutionary.

When I first started, it did not feel fake to me because I was not trying to pretend I was feeling a certain way about a specific situation.

I wasn't thinking about someone I had problems with and trying to make myself feel compassion. Or looking at my bank account and hammering the feeling of safety into my being.

I had done that many times before – and had failed every single time.

But here I was looking at the pure feeling of compassion. I was contemplating the pure feeling of safety. Not applied to my "issues", just "out there in the world".

I did feel it and my mood lifted.

I had to give up thinking about my problems though, that's true. Or I used them as a bouncing place into this new world of pure good feelings.

I will tell you more about what this process did for me in time in the last section, "Living the Goose Bumps".

For now let me just assure you that it works – and that it will "spill over" into your problems too, without any extra effort on your part.

Is it easy to do?

Yes and no.

Like I said before in my food and exercise analogy, if you are used to eating junk food and sitting on the couch, eating healthy food and going for a run will feel utterly uncomfortable.

Doing this more than once will test you to the limit.

And committing to a practice that will really make a difference and completely change your life will... revolutionize your life.

I have found this emotional process to be much the same.

Done a little bit here and there has benefits in and of itself, just like eating one healthy meal and going for one single walk WILL benefit you right then and there – but it will probably change your life.

Do this focusing on pure good feelings for a week and you will start seeing strange things happening. Your "emotional molecules" will start rearranging. Your whole life will start to shift. It is intoxicating – and worth sticking to it.

* * *

There is a second and very important part of this chapter, which I have titled "Cultivate the CLOSEST positive feeling you can reach for."

Let me explain.

Over all the years of living with anxiety and depression I tried many times to "snap out of it" and go for better feelings.

I tried to go from being desperate to being hopeful, or from insecure to confident. Or from powerless to powerful.

And you know what?

I failed!

A lot!

I was reaching for these emotions and one of two things would happen:

1) I would fail to reach them but PRETEND that I did.

Or

2) I would reach them but they would last only a SHORT WHILE.

I never did become the confident person I was reaching for, or the powerful one.

To make matters worse, every time I failed I fell even lower – because now I was disappointed with myself and with life itself.

It wasn't until I started cultivating feelings on purpose that I had this revelation:

IT IS A LOT EASIER TO CONJURE OR CALL IN A LOW-ENERGY FEELING THAN A HIGH-ENERGY ONE WHEN WE ARE STARTING FROM THE NEGATIVE.

In other words, the bigger the "gap" between your current emotional state and your desired one, the harder it is to jump over it (or build a bridge, if you will) – if not impossible.

THE HAPPINESS SWITCH

THIS is WHY efforts to change or shift who you are on a habitual basis fail!

You are trying to do too much, jump too high.

You can't go from the basement in one fell swoop to the top floor in the emotional world, any more than you can do it in the physical world!

You need to start small.

In the next section I will show you how to do that.

Before we do though, I want to tell you one more thing: at the end of the book, in Appendix B, you can find a short reference list of positive feelings ranked in the order of "power", from the mildest to the most powerful.

You can use it as a starting point in your explorations of good feelings, or whenever you feel stuck and unable to move emotionally.

If you have any experiences you would like to share, or thoughts about how to make this better, please email me at findgoodfeelings@gmail.com. I do read all my mail and respond to every message.

So now let's jump, shall we?

CHRISTINE ELLIS

The Workings of the Emotional Trampoline: Bouncing From the Negative to the Positive

So now you have a better idea about how you feel.

You also know how to cultivate feelings on purpose, at will.

We have also discussed the fact that feelings have different emotional charges or intensities. Curiosity is more charged than neutrality but less than excitement.

Moreover, that it is a lot easier, achievable and long-lasting to make small emotional jumps than to reach for highly-charged feelings right off the bat.

So putting all of these things together and connecting the dots, the process of shifting negative feelings is quite simple.

Bouncing into the good involves two steps:

1) take your emotional temperature

We have looked at that in a previous section. Just sit with yourself and try to give a name to what you are feeling. Is it intensely charged like depressed or angry? Or a bit tamer like bored or annoyed?

The name you give the feeling doesn't even matter so much. The exploration is much more important – and the attention that you give to yourself.

If you need help, you can consult the feelings worksheet that I have included in Appendix A.

2) choose a good feeling that you want to cultivate

instead, which is not too highly charged that you cannot reach it

Let's look at some examples, as this is the best way to show you how this process works for me.

Example #1

Say, for instance, that you feel depressed.

You ask yourself: "What is the easiest good feeling I would like to feel instead?"

There can actually be several answers to that: excitement and enthusiasm come to mind.

But when you feel depressed, those are too highly charged.

You can actually recoil from them, because the emotions are too strong and in opposition to how you feel right now.

Instead, you might try to reach for lesser charged emotions such as **calmness** or **curiosity** that are still opposed to depression but not so highly charged that you cannot reach.

When you feel depressed, focusing on the feeling of curiosity can be a whole lot better.

But even those lower-energy emotions, good as they are, might not work for you.

When you are in the midst of despair the last thing you might want is to tell yourself "Be calm!".

THE HAPPINESS SWITCH

Because depression has a strong component of fear, telling yourself to "be calm" is like yelling at a frightened child to settle down and not fret.

Or you may feel that you just "don't give a c..p" about anything so you are not curious about anything at all.

So don't push yourself. The goal here is to make you feel GOOD, or at least BETTER.

Be gentle with yourself and look for the lowest-energy emotion that you can find and that is appealing to you.

You will know instantly when you have a match because you will feel a sort of pull, or click if you will, as if you've found a piece of the puzzle.

For me, **curiosity** is such a feeling.

Even in the midst of my darkest days and most horrible feelings, curiosity is a feeling that I can reach for.

And no, I don't mean "Get curious about your issues."

I mean curiosity feels good in and of itself.

I might think: "Where does curiosity show itself? Who is curious? About what?"

The answers could be:

- Curiosity shows itself in scientists at work

- Curiosity shows itself in a little kitten exploring a room

- Curiosity shows itself in star-gazers

- Curiosity shows itself in people passionate about learning

- Curiosity is on the face of a little boy who is looking in the window of a bike shop

- Curiosity is in a little girl on the eve of her birthday party

Once I get going, I will actually start feeling better and better just "hanging out with curiosity".

Then, when I feel I have drenched yourself enough in the general feeling of curiosity, I might turn it towards my own life.

I might ask: "What makes me curious? Or who?"

Again, the answers are limitless:

- Curiosity, for me, shows itself in literature. I like reading because I am curious about stories – and their authors.

- Curiosity, for me, shows itself in taking walks in the city. I like seeing what's new in stores.

- Curiosity, for me, shows itself in browsing new releases in film. I want to know what my favorite actors, actresses and directors are up to.

THE HAPPINESS SWITCH

- Curiosity, for me, shows itself in art classes. I am thirsty about this kind of learning.

You can continue as long as you want – or stop after the first one.

I can guarantee that once you get going, it won't be long before you will actually want to start putting this in practice. You WILL want to pick up a book, see a movie or check out a new art class.

The old issue will still be there, along with the cloud of the depression. But it will seem smaller somehow. You will have put your attention on something nourishing instead. You will, so to speak, have eaten emotional broccoli.

Will this one exercise be enough? Probably not. But you can try it again.

You can come back to this again and again and each time you will discover something new.

I get curious about life itself and the physical processes on Planet Earth. YouTube videos are wonderful for that.

Looking for new recipes to cook for my family is another way to get myself interested and curious about something.

I am always, always curious about how my closest friends are doing.

Or I hop on Amazon.com to look for new books to discover,

or new music.

Oh yes, and movies! Movies have never failed me and I don't think they ever will.

You see how this is working?

Within less than five minutes, I have shifted my focus out of "the blues" and into life-giving curiosity.

If you pursue this further, for an hour or two or even a day or two, your mood will totally shift.

I mean, what's better: ruminating or getting curious about something?

Example #2

Sometimes, if the feeling of sadness or powerlessness is very strong, I can't work myself up to curiosity.

I have another feeling that never fails me, which is not very highly charged at all but feels incredibly soothing: comfort.

Even in the throes of the most horrible emotional pain, I can always find at least A LITTLE bit of comfort to focus on.

Again, asking the questions: "Who feels comfortable?" I might come up with answers like:

- a little cat in utter comfort, purring on the knees of her favorite person

THE HAPPINESS SWITCH

- an elephant rolling in the mud

- people laying on the beach with a good book, under an umbrella, sipping a cold drink

Often two or three ideas about animals being comfortable in their dens or nests or whatever are enough to evoke the feeling of comfort in me (animals are much better in their own skins than we are, isn't it?).

So then I look for all the comforts I have in my life – and there are MANY:

- a soft pillow and a warm bed

- nice shower gels (don't laugh, everything counts!)

- my favorite wool blanket

- running water (don't we take this for granted…)

- a decent car

"Comfort" is a go-to feeling for me.

It may not be for you though!

Some people feel guilty about having material comforts. If that's the case for you, then try and reach for something else.

You might even try "neutral"! It will surely slow down the strong negative current of depression.

If you are angry, this might work too!

Just ask yourself: "Where does neutrality show itself in the world? Who feels neutral? About what? When? Why? When do I feel neutral?"

Some of the answers might be:

- I am neutral towards sports. I don't hate them, I'm not crazy about them.

- I am neutral towards the color beige. Again, don't love it but I don't hate it either.

- A car not moving, in neutral

- An elephant towards human TV shows

These are just a few examples and I hope that by now I have given you a clear understanding of what I do.

When I first started this practice of cultivating good feelings on purpose, it took me a while to come up with ideas.

Now I do it all the time.

I have shifted the balance in my head. I used to spend a lot of the time obsessing over the past and worrying about the future, very tense about the present – or worse.

Now I spend a lot of my time thinking about pure good feelings.

THE HAPPINESS SWITCH

I cannot begin to tell you how rewarding this is in and of itself.

The inner demons have been appeased.

And by the way, we still need to talk about what to do when they are not quite going with your program of thinking about flower petals and ice-cream and want you to go back to being tormented.

We will talk about that in the next section.

For now, let me tell you a bit about how my life has changed since I stumbled upon this walking, day-in-and-day-out practice of cultivating good feelings on purpose:

- My nightmares have considerably diminished. While I was struggling with the PTSD, I used to have bad dreams at least twice a week. And when I say "bad", I mean really bad. Now I rarely get them (every few months).

- I am enjoying every day and I wake up eager to start

- I am rarely procrastinating

- All of my relationships have improved and I have no more problems setting limits or saying no

- I have the courage and the follow-through to go after my dreams

- I am much more confident

The inner war is basically over.

Do I still have bad moments? Sure I do. But they are moments, not days, or weeks, or months.

In time my confidence in my ability to turn a bad mood around has increased, which helped decrease the power of the bad mood in and of itself.

I am, in other words, emotionally in shape.

Do I still have scars and stretch marks? Sure.

But who cares about those?!

I can honestly say that I am living goose-bumps moments every single day.

I will tell you more a little bit later about living with the goose-bumps but for now, let's talk a bit more about dealing with a phenomenon that will surely show up: the resistance to change.

Dealing with the Resistance to Change

LOOKING AT THIS FROM OUTSIDE, YOU WOULD THINK THAT a process like this, which has only good things to give you, would be something that the whole of you will embark on with great enthusiasm.

But if you have been on the self-growth path for a while, you know this one truth:

JUST BECAUSE SOMETHING IS GOOD FOR YOU DOESN'T MEAN THAT YOU WILL DO IT.

Sometimes people call this inertia.

When you have gathered a lot of momentum, it is definitely harder to stop. A fast moving car will need more time (and breaking power) to slow down in order to turn.

Also, to continue this moving vehicle analogy, it is better to slow down (way down) before you make a turn.

So why is it that we are so resistant to change?

I am not really sure and to be honest, I'm not even that interested in the answer.

All I want is the result: the change itself.

Sure, there are chemicals that get generated in the human body. What neurobiologist Candice Pert calls "molecules of emotion".

These are real "drugs" that get secreted in your body, when you feel something – good or bad.

You can get (and do!) addicted to thoughts and emotions in the same way that you get addicted to nicotine, alcohol or other drugs!

I don't claim to have the cure for that, but I have found my way out of the negative feelings addiction.

I have already explained to you my method.

But now I want to address what the resistance might look like – and what to do about it. Or at least what those two issues were like for me. You might (and surely will) have different experiences, but you will relate enough to mine that you will understand and know what to do.

There were parts of me that wanted no part of this good feeling stuff.

The way this played out for me was through a very harsh form of internal dialogue that:

- **criticized**

- **ridiculed** the process

- insulted and shamed the process and the part of me that pursued it

- threated to "destroy" happiness, health and progress

I would "hear" comments such as:

"This is stupid. It will never worked."

"You have tried so many times before. Give it up!"

"Who the hell do you think you are? You have discovered a… process?! Pfffff…. Hahahahahhaha!"

"If you continue this way, something REALLY bad will happen (and I can't tell you what it will be, but it will be horrible!).

This and much more.

All of it was very familiar. I'm sure it is to you too, if you have been living with the blues.

So this is what I did about it:

NOTHING.

That's right.

I did NOT fight them and told those "voices" to stop.

I did NOT try to convince.

I did NOT get mad.

I just went on with the business of focusing on the good feelings.

Because when you are deeply absorbed by something, these "voices" stop. Have you noticed?

But I will say this:

The negative voices are louder when you are trying to reach for too much, too fast.

Do you remember how we were talking about the big jump between depression and excitement? Or fear and confidence?

I noticed in time that if I tried to reach for too much, too fast, I would get flooded with messages like the above from the scared and resistant parts of me.

In that sense, they are incredibly useful.

THE HAPPINESS SWITCH

They became a signal to take it all down to an achievable level.

Because they didn't seem that threated by comfort, or neutrality, or indifference or curiosity.

Maybe it is because "they" didn't think that much can be accomplished by focusing on those "measly feelings".

That was my shortcut around those voices that had prevented me so many times before from making real and lasting change.

What happens after a while though is that the chemical balance in your body LITERALLY changes.

I would imagine that the same thing happened after I quit smoking. For a while, I could still taste the nicotine in my mouth and I had the strong cravings. In time, the taste went away.

Strangely enough, the cravings stayed much longer than the after-taste.

I won't discuss here why that is. It doesn't even matter.

What matters is that if you get hooked on the really good stuff, the well-being feelings, the ones that give you life instead of sucking it out of you, the chemistry of your body changes.

When the balance gets tipped, you will find yourself thinking good thoughts without making an effort.

I will talk about that more in the section called "Living the Goose Bumps".

For now, just know that is it possible. Not only that, but it is entirely achievable – in a relatively short amount of time.

How much time?

That depends on you, really.

If you stick with it, you will see results within days. They will motivate you to keep going so within a matter of weeks, your life can completely transform.

But I have a few warnings to give you.

This process is delicate and you need a soft hand with it.

In part III I will tell you exactly what I mean by that.

Before we move on, let's do a quick recap – and what I call an a-ha exercise.

A Brief Recap

SO FAR I HAVE TAUGHT YOU EVERYTHING I HAVE DEVELOPED so far in what I call "The Good Feelings Method", specifically applied to anxiety, depression and other low-energy states.

In its shortest version, the process has two steps:

1) Taking your emotional temperature (knowing where you are)

And

2) Choosing the closest positive feeling available to you and cultivating it.

To put all the fine points where they need to be, we need to further add that the bigger the jump between feelings, the harder it is to make (and stay in the higher state!). In other words, you won't be able to jump from depression to excitement. But you could go from depression to curiosity or comfort.

This is why I say that you need to choose the closest positive feeling available to you.

As for cultivating a specific feeling, this simply means looking around to see where it appears –who feels it and in what circumstances.

The idea here is that simply by watching it and recognizing it in others, you are feeling it yourself.

It may not be applied to the specific situations of your own life – in fact, it is recommended that you start (and stay) with pure feelings for a while.

You will literally rewire your circuits, change the chemistry in your body and start different circuits in your brain that will grow stronger and stronger the more you do this.

Your life will change because you will not only have more inner resources to deal with it, but the good feelings that you will cultivate are attractive in nature in and of themselves.

Happy people attract happy life circumstances and unhappy people... well, you know how that one goes.

Is this a cure?

> *"The world breaks everyone and afterward many are strong in the broken places."* **Ernest Hemingway**

SOMETIMES PEOPLE ASK ME IF I BELIEVE THAT DEPRESSION can be cured. Or anxiety. Or whatever other name you want to give to states that basically mean "not thriving and not well".

There are some who would answer emphatically NO.

My answer would be... it depends what your definition of a cure is.

I have used the food analogy a lot so far. I would like to stay with it a bit more so I can explain what I mean.

Say you are overweight and that, in time, you manage to pack on quite a few pounds.

It is making you miserable in every possible way (or is it the other way around, as in you got that way because you were feeling miserable?! Whichever it is, you now want to change – both your weight and your thinking).

You decide that you will do the two obvious things that people do when they want to lose weight:

- eating healthy foods and in smaller quantities

- moving your body.

The first few days (or weeks or even months) the change will not be easy. Not at all.

Depending on how you are build (personality, body chemistry etc.) and your personal history (traumas etc.) you might have a really hard time.

Some people have nightmares for months. Others live with panic attacks during the day.

Change is scary - and can be really, really hard.

But you stick to it because you know that it works. Others have done it, you have seen the results.

So in time it gets easier. You start losing the weight. You huff and puff less when you are going for a run, a swim or whatever ways of moving your body you chose.

THE HAPPINESS SWITCH

There comes a time when you are very close to your desired goal: your ideal weight.

By then many things will have changed: you might be getting attention from the opposite sex and now you have to deal with THAT anxiety (it can be scary being in the limelight!); some of your friendships might dissolve because of jealousy or lack of common interests; you are getting more assertive at work because you are more confident, since you have accomplished such a big feat as changing your body and your emotions.

But does this really mean that you never have bad days? That you never overeat? That you don't have scars on your body that show its former state? Or that you never again fall into old emotional patterns from time to time?

Probably not.

It's just that the proportion has changed: instead of feeling bad most of the time and good every once in a while, now you feel good a lot. The bad moments are much less frequent – and now you know what to do about them.

You are wise enough to let the storm pass.

So you are well again. Now you have a way of being in the world that you can count on.

Would you call this a cure? I for one would say yes.

Part III: Easy Does It (and why it is really, really, really important that you do!)

1. A Cautionary Tale

I HAVE GIVEN THIS SECTION THE TITLE "A Cautionary Tale". It sounds a bit dramatic and I don't mean to scare you... but I do want to tell you that this stuff really does work.

This focusing on feelings, which evokes feelings in you, is powerful alchemy. It is powerful magic.

You may think, as they do in fairy tales, that all magic comes with a price. Well, you can think of it that way.

There is a price. But not in the way you think.

At least it wasn't like I had pictured it for me.

Not that I was imagining bad witches flying in from other planets ready to curse me, or a vengeful G-d chasing after me for chanting in front of a white candle...

But something did happen to me that brought it spookily close to magic – and all the warnings that are given whenever you perform such feats.

They all do say "Proceed with caution."

I had to pay the price and learn from my own experience what they meant, because it really wasn't just blah-blah.

I'll tell you a bit more of my own story to illustrate this point.

I have already told you in the beginning of this book how I started on this journey of cultivating pure feelings.

I have shared with you my own dramas and traumas, my struggles and issues.

Now that I have shared my road to emotional success, so to speak, you have an even better idea of where I started and where I am right now.

I want to share one more episode with you.

When my son was a little over a year old I decided I had enough. I was going to keep an "appreciation" journal and write in it all the good things that happened during the day.

THE HAPPINESS SWITCH

Darn it, I was gonna do it! I was gonna rid myself of "negativity" once and for all.

So every night I wrote down at least ten things to be "grateful" for that had happened that day. You know, like they teach you in all the gratitude books. Write about waking up in the morning. Write about your hair. Write about your cat. Write about a yummy dish. Write about your full tummy.

If I sound a bit bitter, it's because I am. You see, this "gratitude" thing didn't really work for me. Even while I was doing it, I did so through gritted teeth. I still felt tension and anxiety. It did nothing to change my anxiety. I was simply beating myself over the head with the "gratitude pole", as if saying to myself "Hey you ungrateful dummy, who can't you appreciate instead of feeling afraid? Just STOP your whining and APPRECIATE!"

Three months later I ran a brand new car into an electricity pole. I still can't explain how it happened exactly. I was on a small country road and the car was moving very slowly, I looked at the dashboard for what felt like a few second and the next thing I knew, I was in the ditch, heading for the pole.

Oh and no, I saw no miracles during those three months of forced nightly gratitude. My life didn't change and neither did my fear and anxiety.

But back to that day when I crashed the car for the first time in my life… everyone was fine and I came out of it shaken but determined to do two things:

1) stop pushing so hard against myself

2) get really serious about it and find a way to be good with myself that worked for me.

Because... clearly this "moving of energy" was working. I had moved it enough with my "gratitude" in order to manifest THAT. But why hadn't all the "appreciation" worked in my favor? How come I "manifested" a car crash?

Scared and confused, I took things slowly. At first I wanted to understand.

I sat with my fear and the facts of what had happened and at some point I had a flash of insight: I had not been going TOWARDS the things I wanted, I was RUNNING AWAY from depression, financial loss and "all bad things".

It only seemed as if I was looking towards the "good things" but really, I was staring fear in the face and hoping joy would show up like a far-away angel. So fear grew. I was growing it every night, when I put down on paper all the good things, but saying in fact "Whew! I've avoided you today – fear, depression and all my old friends."

It started to make sense.

So then... I gave up the struggle. I gave up the determination. That's what had gotten me into the pole, in the name of "appreciation".

I just sort of took it easy and started to look at "general things".

THE HAPPINESS SWITCH

The key point that I want to make here is that "Easy does it!" is not a phrase for the weak. It is the way of life for the powerful wizard! This is why they say that the master has ease. Ease is a prerequisite though.

Whenever you feel yourself starting to push, STOP! Take a break. Go get a glass of water or, even better, back off the subject until you don't feel so tensed, so "darn determined" anymore.

And no, I am not knocking down gratitude and appreciation. I am simply saying that they need to come naturally. It's a bit like falling in love – the more you try to push yourself on someone, the more they back off. You have to let things happen naturally.

Gratitude and appreciation will develop naturally as your life will gradually start changing for the better, as your fear will diminish and as you will be more and more comfortable in your skin.

Don't fall for the trap of urgency and the scares that fear builds inside your head.

If you are dealing with explosives, you'd better do it gently. It's sort of the same here.

The other thing is, I'm not knocking determination either. But there is a good kind, which makes people follow "impossible" goals to fruition, sometimes through years or decades of trying.

There's also a bad kind, which grits people's teeth and makes them obsess. Whenever there's a "Darn it!" screaming inside of you, stop and take a breath. See which kind of determination you are following.

If you are gritting your teeth, it is the wrong kind. If this hits you, please STOP, take a break! Regroup and rest in this idea, even if you don't fully believe it:

EVERYTHING IS ALRIGHT

Go see a movie or take a warm bath or go for a walk and give it a rest. Learn something new, bake a cake, sand and paint an old table... whatever it is that you enjoy doing.

Don't give in to a false sense of urgency. It will not lead you to good places.

Sometimes this is hard to do, I know. When you feel like you have a burning issue, the world teaches you to plough ahead in full force.

But dealing with emotions is much like dealing with electricity: you really need to know what you are doing in order to harness it.

It will come. Remind yourself that and soothe yourself just like you would a frightened child.

Tomorrow you will start again.

2. Baby Steps

IN THIS CHAPTER I WILL CONTINUE THE THEME of "Easy Does It" with a practical way to put that in action: namely, baby steps.

We all like dramatic turnarounds, huge jumps and fast achievements. But the truth is, life needs a slower pace in order to develop. Things take time. And they grow a little bit at a time.

If you are in pain, you want quick and immediate relief. You can have that in the form of a pill – or a shot of alcohol – but the deeper and underlying issue probably needs more than that.

As tempting as a quick "win" might seem, don't fall for it. Allow yourself to take baby steps. Sooner than you think, they will add up to make you realize you have completely changed your course.

For example, if you are feeling depressed and discouraged, don't try to jump to excitement and enthusiasm. It's too big of a jump. You may succeed for a while, but it won't last.

Instead, reach for "lower key" feelings – which are, in fact, incredibly powerful in bringing about change. One of those feelings is curiosity. Instead of despondency, cultivate interest. In anything. It will completely shift your mood.

3. Imperfect is Perfectly Fine

DON'T WORRY ABOUT GETTING EVERYTHING RIGHT. Don't worry about doing anything perfectly.

Beating down on ourselves is the main reason why we end up in the dumps anyway.

And we beat down on ourselves primarily because we find all kinds of crazy reasons why what we do and how we live are not PERFECT. We have learned it somewhere along the way, from a parent or someone "REALLY important". Even if we get it right one blessed day, it's still not good enough because "Can you do it again? Soon?"

When it comes to emotions, nothing ever need be perfect. Everything is changing anyway. We cannot bottle moments of perfect emotion to keep them forever. We must learn how to allow them to happen over and over again. This is what this course is about.

So it is worth saying that simply showing up, in your mind, is a really big deal.

It is worth saying that catching yourself heading towards a negative spiral is a really big deal. You don't even have to turn it around. Just seeing it is huge.

It is worth saying that love and kindness are as far away from perfection as you can possibly imagine. They can and are, in and of themselves, perfect for they are the highest vibration of the heart. But they do not require the struggle, the pain and the straight-jacket of perfectionism.

So kick off your shoes and let yourself just FEEL.

4. Put One Feeling Before the Other

YOU DO KNOW THAT SAYING: "PUT ONE FOOT in front of the other" – and its cousin "The thousand miles journey starts with a single step." Here they very much apply.

You are embarking on a self-directed emotional journey. Nobody, by the way, can do it for you because nobody can feel for you.

Which is why, as a side note, helping others doesn't always

work no matter how hard you try: because you cannot feel good instead of themselves feeling good for themselves, no matter how genuine your desire to help. But I digress...

Let's go back to the emotional journey and the very real need to pace yourself and to not try and do too much in one step, before you get strong enough.

Just like on a physical journey (and boy, have I mixed my metaphors in this book! But I'm not sorry about that because I think it gets my point across), when you start on an emotional journey to feel better and better and then ultimately good, you need to:

-   Gather your supplies. Food, water and good shoes in the case of hiking, a list of good emotions and a method for cultivating them consistently in the case of feeling good.

-   Start small. You wouldn't try to do 10 miles in your first day of a hike. Likewise, you can't expect to feel elation or ecstasy when you start in the pits of despair. A little bit of calmness or curiosity about a little something are much better targets.

I cannot stress enough the importance of starting small – and continuing to take small steps, even when you do get stronger. Even if you manage to cultivate – and consistently feel, during your day – a feeling of serenity, don't jump into feeling joy or elation right away. Go for something in between, like satisfaction or pleasure.

This is what I think of as building your emotional muscles. One small stretch at a time.

THE HAPPINESS SWITCH

I also want to say that many of us (if not most) who suffer or have suffered from anxiety, depression and the other less-than-pleasant emotions for years do have moments of elation and excitement. But those do not last! Not even the short-lived feeling of well-being, of simply feeling good in our skin doesn't last. We get on manic highs that we cannot sustain – because we do not have the emotional stamina to do so. Our emotional muscles are starved and untrained, quite atrophied maybe so how could they last in a high-intensity state?

They can't. So we have yo-yo bounces from the depths of despair to the manic highs.

What I have discovered and am teaching you here is a way to build emotional stamina every single day, moment by moment, in a gentle and kind way.

You may think that this doesn't add up to much – but you try it for a week and see what happens!

Part IV: Living the Goose Bumps

1. Cultivate Potatoes Before You Move on to Orchids

IN THE PREVIOUS CHAPTER I'VE TALKED ABOUT CULTIVATING feelings. I've touched upon this several times in previous lectures. If I sound as if I'm repeating myself, it's because... well, I'm repeating myself. But there is a reason: repetition is how we learn things. Having things explained in many ways and from many angles is how we understand things. At least that's how it works for me – and for my students.

If you've got it the first time around, sit back and enjoy. But I hope you will do the exercises that come with each new lecture.

And now, let me repeat myself some more – in a new way. I've told you before how important it is to start small. I'll say it again: start small. Don't go for ecstasy right off the bat, go for curiosity and giggles.

Now let me say it in a different way: cultivate potatoes before you move on to orchids.

What I mean by this is that when you start gardening, you should begin with the easiest plant you can get your hands on and learn how to put it in the ground, water it properly and pull out the weeds around it – or whatever else it needs in order to grow and flourish.

It is the same with the garden of your mind and the emotions seeds that you want to plant.

The low-voltage ones are easier to cultivate because they are more stable. They have more staying power. They are meant to be that way. Nobody can live in a state of continuous excitement. We'd fry our circuits really fast.

The high-voltage emotions are more volatile. Harder to "catch", in a sense, because they are flying faster. They are not meant to be lived in all the time.

So when you are first starting to cultivate feelings, go for the low-voltage one first.

THE HAPPINESS SWITCH

Low-voltage, by the way, does in no way mean inferior.

We prize high-speed and go for the drama and the shock value in most everything. But life thrives in stability and continuity, in comfort and tenderness, in giggles and simplicity.

So start small. And start simple.

With this lecture I am including a worksheet with a few low-voltage emotions that I have begun sprouting for you. I am inviting you to continue caring for them by contemplating them and "hanging out" with them. I am more than confident that they will give you an amazing crop – and much sooner than you think.

2. A Daily Practice

I HAVE TAUGHT YOU EVERYTHING I KNOW about sorting out your feelings and cultivating happiness on purpose, in the form of the positive emotions that make happiness up: calm, curiosity, comfort, joy, passion, excitement and so on.

By now I hope you know what to do when you are feeling less than good.

But when we say happiness we think of it as something that we want to feel all the time. Or most of the time. We want to minimize the times when we feel bad – and we want to minimize their intensity.

THE HAPPINESS SWITCH

As you know, I define happiness as the sum total of what I feel on a daily basis. Happiness is made of many feelings of different intensities, that flash through me at different times.

So to feel happy all the time (or most of the time), it follows that I need to feel these good feelings a lot. I don't need to feel like bouncing off the walls all the time! In fact, that is neither desirable nor advisable (circuits overload?).

But I do need to cultivate good feelings.

It is a very easy thing to do really, once you understand it. You can do it at any time: in traffic, doing housework, walking your dog, taking a shower. You can even do it while other people are present!

If you don't believe me, think of all the times you have been ruminating over something that is bothering you WHILE you are talking to others. It is exactly the same... only in reverse.

Instead of ruminating, you are contemplating goodness, beauty and love in their many forms.

You can do this on purpose (and I highly recommend that you do) and you can of course do it when you hit some troubled waters.

In a very short time – I am talking about weeks, if not days – your entire mood will shift.

I will tell you what happened to me:

- I learned to shift anxiety and fear.

- I can fully appreciate and savor the people in my life.

- I can fully appreciate and savor my life.

- I have built the emotional stamina to outgrow procrastination. This, in turn, allowed me to finally take action in the direction of my dreams. Which in turn cascaded into many positive and life-giving things, such as growing my blog, my practice and my bank account.

- I am no longer stuck in downward spirals, for days, weeks or months. I know what to do to turn things around.

- I have built the emotional stamina to deal with difficult people in my life – in my own head and without the need for confrontation (which always made things worse). Side note: the funny thing is, when they stopped bothering me "in my head", they stopped being so difficult in real life.

I am far from being a master at it though. I still consider myself a "beginner gardener of emotions". But I love what I am seeing already.

This is a practice that, in the end, is highly specific to YOU. I have given you the framework, but how it plays out in your life is up to you. I hope you put it in practice!

Good emotions are everywhere. Spot them! For when you do, they run through your veins too!

When you go to the park, take in the playfulness of children and dogs and you will feel playful too. Take in the freshness of the leaves and the grass and this will make you feel

THE HAPPINESS SWITCH

refreshed. Take a moment to appreciate a break in your day and the rest that it gives you and you will feel more rested.

Feeling good, like beauty, is in the eyes of the beholder. You can be in the exact same situation and find reasons to feel less than good – of only for ruminating about your work, relationships or whatever.

The garden of the mind stretches far and wide. Cultivate it well. Now you know how.

3. "Build it and they will come".

I HAVE GIVEN THIS CHAPTER THE TITLE "Build it and they will come". I am sure you have heard this expression and you are familiar with its meaning.

In the business world it means "Build the structure/business/idea before you have any customers – and then the customers will come".

The expression was made popular by an American movie called "Field of Dreams" in which the main character, played by Kevin Costner, builds a baseball field in the hopes that if it is there, people will show up to watch baseball. And they do.

THE HAPPINESS SWITCH

Of course, there is more to it than that, but at the end of the movie Kevin Costner's character does get his wish. People come to watch baseball being played on a field he had built for that.

I think that we apply this in many ways in our lives. We go to school, for example, before we have a specific job in mind. We prepare ourselves for a romantic relationship before we meet someone we like.

The goal is not very clear and many times it is far in the future, but we start "building" anyway, because we know that if we do, it will happen.

It is much the same in the world of feelings.

If you build your emotional garden on positive feelings, this will generate positive thoughts which in turn will lead you to positive actions. All combined will create not only a happy life, but I am willing to bet it will be extraordinary too.

The feelings you cultivate are, as we have already discussed, attractive in nature. They are magnetic. They "pull in" whatever it is on a similar wavelength.

If you "build" pathways of serenity, you will have peaceful relationships, a calm home, smooth life circumstances, to give you a few examples.

If you "build" pathways of joy, you will have interesting work, a lot of fun with friends and family and awesome vacations – to give you a few more examples.

Of course, it will not all be perfect. Of course, things won't always go as planned. Of course you will have the occasional slump, bad day and crappy mood. But you will have a strong foundation for good, and good will prevail.

So don't wait until your life is "going well" or even "going better". Start cultivating good feelings NOW.

Closing Words

We have reached the end of this book, but I sincerely hope that this is not the end of our journey together.

I have created an online course based on the material I have presented to you here.

It has video lectures, more good feelings video meditations and many more a-ha exercises. Please do check it out.

You can also sign up for my updates at **www.findgoodfeelings.wordpress.com**. I will be sending you free video meditations, books and courses from other authors that I like and whose work impacts my life, as well as discounts and promotions.

You can find a community of like-minded people by joining my Facebook Group.

I really hope hearing from you and your progress and I sincerely hope that you will keep me posted.

I will celebrate with you every step of the way.

Till we meet again,

Christine

Appendix A

NEGATIVE FEELINGS / EMOTIONS

Afraid

Alarmed

Alone

Angry

Annoyed

Anxious

Ashamed

Bitter

Boiling

Bored

Cold

Cowardly

Crushed

Deprived

Desperate

Diminished

Disappointed

Discouraged

Doubtful

Embarrassed

Empty

Enraged

Fearful

Forced

Frightened

Frustrated

Fuming

Grieved

Guilty

THE HAPPINESS SWITCH

Hateful

Heartbroken

Hesitant

Hostile

Humiliated

Hurt

Indecisive

Indifferent

Inferior

Infuriated

Irritated

Lonely

Lost

Miserable

Nervous

Offended

Panicked

Pathetic

Perplexed

Pessimistic

Powerless

Provoked

Rejected

Resentful

Restless

Sad

Scared

Shy

Skeptical

Sore

Sorrowful

Suspicious

Tense

Terrified

Threatened

Tortured

Uneasy

THE HAPPINESS SWITCH

Unhappy

Unpleasant

Unsure

Upset

Useless

Victimized

Vulnerable

Worried

Wronged

POSITIVE FEELINGS / EMOTIONS

Absorbed

Accepting

Admired

Admiring

Adored/adoring

Affectionate

Alive

Amazed

Amused

Animated

Attentive

Attracted

Attractive

Aware

Awe

Balanced

Beautiful

THE HAPPINESS SWITCH

Blessed

Blissful

Blooming

Bold

Brave

Breathtaking

Bright

Calm

Capable

Captivated

Celebrated

Certain

Charming

Cheered

Cheerful

Cherished

Clever

Close

Colorful

Comfortable

Comforted

Confident

Connected

Considerate

Consistent

Content

Creative

Curious

Daring

Dazzling

Delighted

Determined

Decided

Dedicated

Desired/Desirable

Devoted

THE HAPPINESS SWITCH

Dynamic

Eager

Earnest

Easy

Ecstatic

Effective

Efficient

Elated

Embraced

Empowered

Enchanted

Encouraged

Energetic

Entertained

Enthusiastic

Excited

Exhilarated

Expansive

Expressive

Exuberant

Fabulous

Familiar

Fantastic

Fascinated/Fascinating

Feminine

Festive

Fit

Flexible

Flourishing

Flowing

Focused

Fond of

Fortunate

Free

Frisky

Fulfilled

THE HAPPINESS SWITCH

Fun

Generous

Gentle

Gifted

Giggly

Glad

Glamorous

Gleeful

Glowing

Graceful

Grounded

Guided

Happy

Harmonious

High

Hopeful

Imaginative

Immense

Important

Impressive

Impressed

Improved

Infinite

Influential

Innocent

Innovative

Inquisitive

Insightful

Inspired

Inspiring

Interested

Interesting

Intrigued

Intuitive

Inviting

Joyful

Joyous

THE HAPPINESS SWITCH

Jubilant

Keen

Kind

Light

Lovable

Loved

Loving

Lovely

Lucky

Lush

Luxurious

Magical

Magnetic

Mesmerizing

Natural

Neutral

Nice

Neat

Optimistic

Organized

Overjoyed

Passionate

Peaceful

Perceptive

Playful

Pleased

Plentiful

Poetic

Positive

Powerful

Praised

Precise

Profound

Progressive

Provocative

Pure

Quiet

THE HAPPINESS SWITCH

Reassured

Rebellious

Receptive

Refreshed

Relaxed

Reliable

Relieved

Resourceful

Rested

Restored

Rich

Romantic

Safe

Satisfied

Secure

Sensitive

Sensual

Serene

Shiny

Significant

Simple

Sincere

Skilled

Smooth

Sparkly

Special

Spirited

Splendid

Stable

Stimulated

Stimulating

Strong

Sublime

Subtle

Successful

Sumptuous

Sunny

THE HAPPINESS SWITCH

Superb

Supported

Sweet

Sympathetic

Synchronized

Talented

Tenacious

Tender

Thrilled

Touched

Touching

Tranquil

Treasured

Triumphant

Trusted

Trusting

Truthful

Understanding

Understood

Unique

Unstoppable

Valuable

Valued

Varied

Vast

Vigorous

Visionary

Vital

Warm

Warmed

Wealthy

Welcomed

Wise

Wonderful

Worthy

Young

Youthful

APPENDIX B

A SHORT LIST OF POSITIVE FEELINGS / EMOTIONS RANKED IN THE ORDER OF THEIR "CHARGE"

Neutral

Calm

Comfortable

Gentle

Peaceful

Satisfied

Curious

Intrigued

Harmonious

Encouraged

Capable

Eager

Connected

Affectionate

Wise

Kind

Enchanted

Energetic

Excited

Blooming

Giggly

Playful

Inspired

Passionate

Wonderful

Elated

THE HAPPINESS SWITCH

Exhilarated

Blissful

Triumphant

The Companion Workbook

I have created a short, to-the-point companion workbook for the material in this book.

It contains a few exercises based on what we have discussed, in order to help you and guide you in taking control of your feelings.

You can download it free of charge at this address: http://eepurl.com/cnF415.

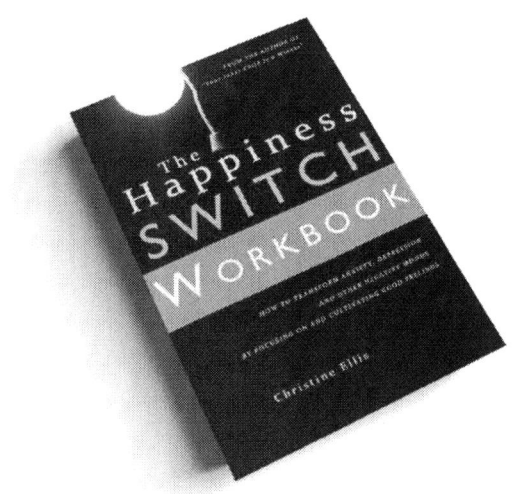

THE HAPPINESS SWITCH

About The Author

CHRISTINE ELLIS is a former teacher who discovered, after being diagnosed with depression and PTSD, a lasting way to transform her life each and every day: focusing on good feelings.

She now writes books and designs online courses about good feelings and feeling good.

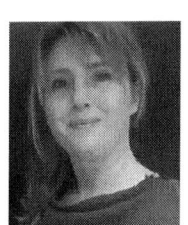

Christine lives in Brussels, Belgium with her husband and young son. All of her stories have a happy ending.

Email: findgoodfeelings@gmail.com.

Visit the Amazon Author Page for the complete list of titles.

https://www.amazon.com/author/christineellis

PLEASE REVIEW

Please leave a review, to help others benefit from the content of this book. Thank you for your support!

THE HAPPINESS SWITCH

Printed in Great Britain
by Amazon